A Simple Guide to the Forefoot Step
Forefoot Step
– Natural walking

AF288302

Dirk Beckmann

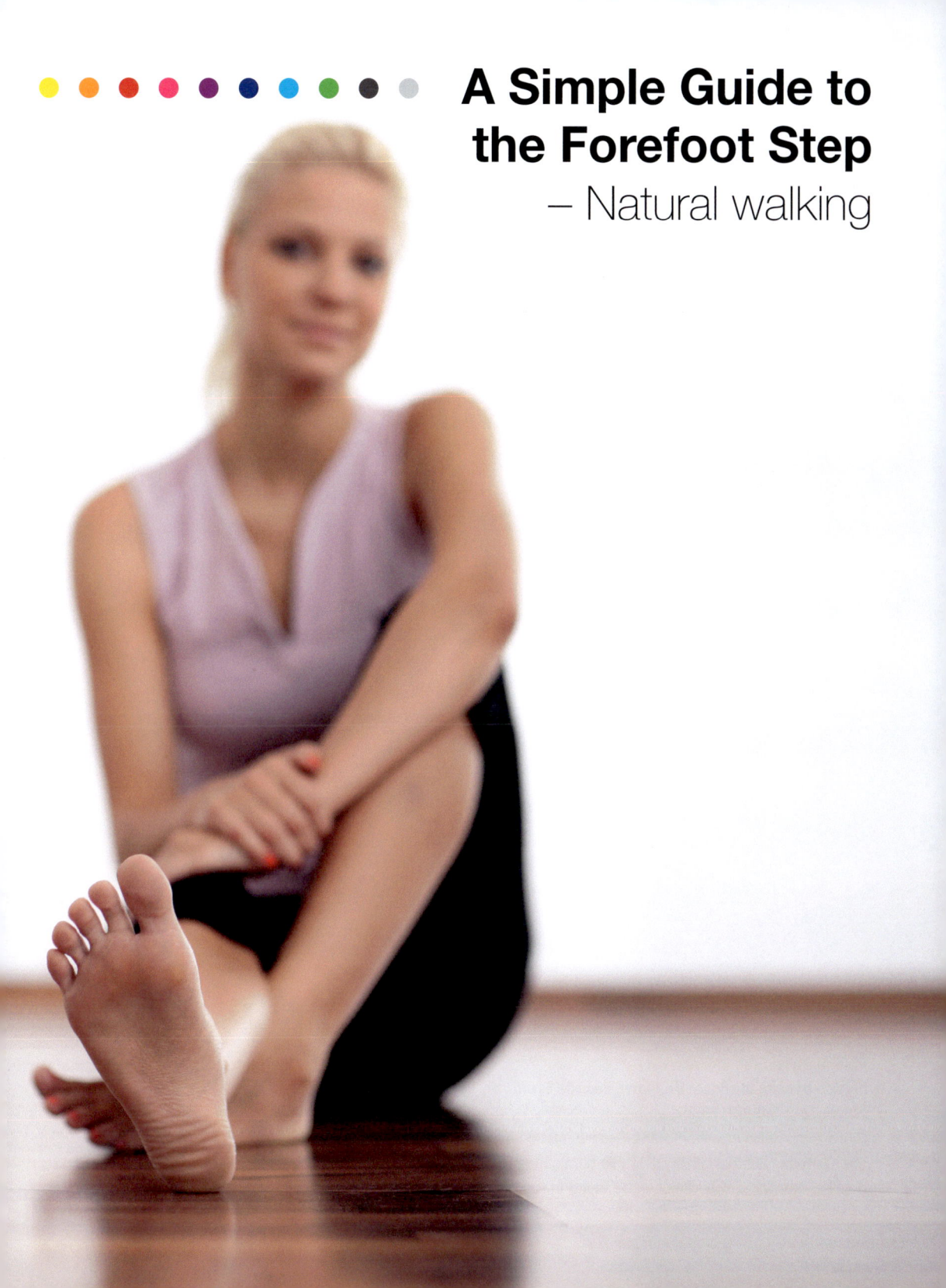

A Simple Guide to the Forefoot Step
– Natural walking

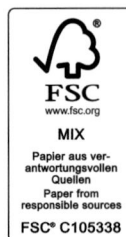

© 2011 Dirk Beckmann

Production and Publishing: Books on Demand GmbH, Norderstedt

Photography: Frank Altmann

English translation: Janet Brümmer, Jessica Brümmer, Terri Dörrzapf

ISBN 978-3-8423-2176-2

Bibliographical information of the German National Library (DNB):

The German National Library lists this publication in the German National Bibliography;

detailed bibliographical data can be found in the Internet at http://dnb.dnb.de.

A Simple Guide to the Forefoot Step
– Natural walking

Foreword

"You've got to roll your feet! Your heel should touch down first on the floor. Then you roll your foot along the outer edge, over the outer and inner ball of the foot and then off over the toes."

In this or a similar manner, dear reader, it has probably been explained to you thousands of times throughout your life how to make things "run smoothly" and walk correctly. (Actually, you need a shoe that acts as a prosthesis for this gait pattern, but more on that later.) There are many books out there on the topic of "proper running", "proper jogging" and so forth. Books about "correct walking", however, are quite rare, even though walking is probably our most common way of getting around. Just as we speak of "walking upright" as being typical for humans and not "running upright". Whether right is always right will be another subject of this book because I would like to tag 99% of these theories as downright false. Of course you can make up your own mind, and please don't believe me blindly. In this guidebook, I will try to give you an understanding of how the forefoot step works without boring you with the vague theories of countless studies. At the end of the day, it's important to deliver proof, which I would like to do together with you, on the following pages. Additionally I want to get you moving, because as the saying goes, nothing ventured, nothing gained or as athletes like to put it: "no pain, no gain".

As mentioned before, not a lot of good literature can be found on the topic of the forefoot step. I will make references here and there to what I believe are the two main sources on this topic. Dr. Peter Greb, for one, who has been presenting the subject of the forefoot step to an open-minded audience since 1979 and who is a pioneer in this field. Or Frank W. Demann, who, in his own unique way, links the subject of the forefoot step to a functional system of body integration with his Senmotic blue and Senmotic red methods. Although when you think about it, we are actually all experts on walking with a forefoot step, because we all took our first steps this way when we were little.

Contrary to other publications I have read, I will try to give you step-by-step instructions to help you better understand how the forefoot step works on the basis of exercises, which you can practice on your own. However, I do advise you to talk to an expert about forefoot walking, because sometimes getting back on the right track can be a long and exhausting process. The road to success here, in comparison, is anything but mysterious and difficult. All you sometimes have to do is ask for directions.

On the following pages you'll find out why we even need to discuss the subject of what I like to call "the forefoot step", why we don't actually roll along the soles of our feet when we walk, and how to find your way back to the forefoot step. At the end of the book you will also find a couple of tips on how to choose the right shoes for you.

Are you ready? Good, then follow me to the next step.

Forefoot vs. rearfoot – what is this all about?

In the following chapter I want to begin to give you an understanding of the forefoot step and compare it to the so-called rearfoot or heel strike, with which many people are probably more familiar.

When as toddlers we first discovered the gait pattern typical for humans and switched from the horizontal (crawling) to the vertical (standing/walking/running), the forefoot step was instinctively our first choice. We humans have been taking our first steps in this same way for thousands of years: using the forefoot step! The so-called "stepping reflex" of infants is also characterized by a distinctive forefoot step, even long before those first real steps are taken. To test this reflex, the infant is supported underneath its arms and held with its feet just above the floor. When the soles of the feet come in contact with a flat surface, the infant automatically makes small treading movements, touching down first with the ball of the foot and not the heel.

Observing this reflex gave Dr. Greb the idea to develop his Godo® method of forefoot walking. This reflex usually disappears before the age of three months. It's interesting to note that the stepping reflex is included in the so-called "primitive reflexes" exhibited by infants in the initial stages of development. According to this definition, these reflexes occur without any voluntary cerebral involvement. They serve as a primary instinct used for the gathering and ingestion of food or for general self-survival. It's also interesting that with ongoing development of the cerebrum – the part of the brain responsible for conscious thinking, among others – these reflexes are suppressed by "superior functions". At least that is how they are referred to in the field of traditional medicine.

Therefore, on a subconscious level our organism appears to prefer the forefoot step because even after the "stepping reflex" has disappeared, we still learn to walk taking our first steps using the forefoot step technique. At this stage of life a toddler doesn't actively choose the forefoot step over heel striking or, for that matter, any other walking patterns. At such a tender age we simply use the most efficient way of walking available to us. The program we already have installed on our hard drives, so to speak. And with good reason. Let's take a closer look at another example:

As a therapist specializing in muscles and fascia (dense connective tissue that gives structure to your body) I make my living helping people rebalance their bodies. This is combined with an increase in mobility and an improvement of upright body posture. The person becomes "more aligned". Now take a look at toddlers who are just taking their first steps or are standing up alone for the first time. You will notice very quickly that these little people stand and sit up very straight. Their heads seem to balance exactly above their small bodies with no apparent effort. Why does something that comes so easily to toddlers cause us grown-ups such problems, often even pain? Well, take a look around you. How many people do you see every day who slouch with their heads leaning forward, twisted or slanted sideways? Don't bother counting because I can tell you: there are a lot! And believe me I know, because thanks to the more intelligent of these contemporaries who are also ready to make a change, I am able to bring home the bacon for my family.

So what is different during early childhood? Well, as babies our muscles are just strong enough to allow us to move. The strength of the neck and back muscles is not yet developed enough to hold up the head – which, in proportion to the body, is huge – either in front of the body or in a non-balanced position. The same goes for the muscle chains of the entire body. If the toddler carried its head as far forward as your neighbor, the woman in the tram or your boss, the baby would simply topple over on its face.

As a grown adult, on the other hand, you have enough energy reserves to compensate such false posture – with all the resulting muscle imbalances and afflictions. Because taking on a battle against gravity takes some effort. Quite a lot of effort actually, even though only few people are aware of this. And your chances of winning the battle against the omnipresent force of gravity are extremely slim. Let's say they equal zero because time is also on gravity's side. The toddler on the other hand adapts to gravity so skillfully that a minimum of effort is required to remain upright because that is the amount of energy at its disposal. Or have you ever seen such a small human being fighting against gravity by tensing up its stomach and buttocks?

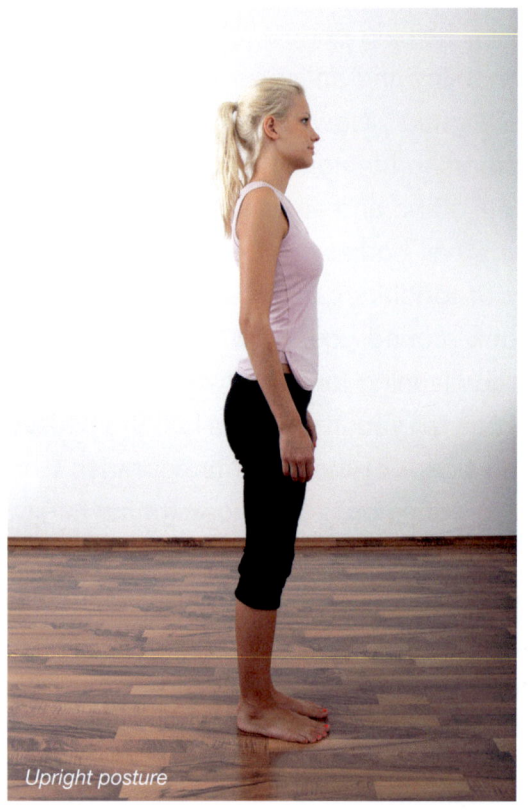

Upright posture

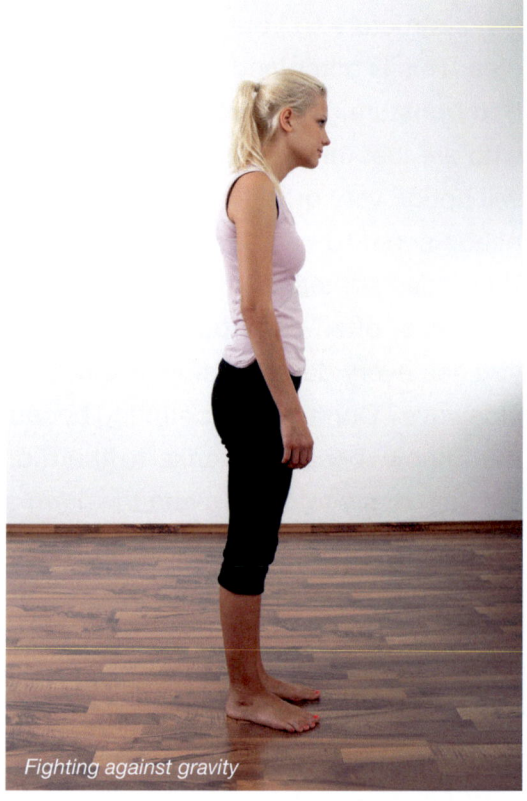

Fighting against gravity

Likewise these little people automatically adopt the most efficient pattern when it comes to walking and this has always been the forefoot step. Interestingly enough, you, too, constantly use the forefoot step without even wondering about it. I know you might be reading these statements with slightly raised eyebrows now. You don't believe me? Just stand up and check how good you already are at implementing the forefoot step!

How do you use your feet, for instance, when walking backwards?

Interesting, isn't it? You land on the forefoot before bringing down the heel. But let's not stop there. What is it like when you walk sideways? Hey, how about that! Again the forefoot! Which part of your foot do you use when going up stairs and which part when going down stairs? Interesting, isn't it? It's the forefoot. And how about when dancing up and down like Muhammad Ali, one moment as light-footed as a butterfly, then stinging powerfully like a bee the next? What can I say? Again, you're prancing on the balls of your feet. Dancing is a good cue here, because in familiar standard dances and many folk dances all over the world people mainly move in a forefoot stepping pattern. What is it like when we sprint? You'll notice here as well that the heels of the world's fastest runners never even touch the ground when they sprint. Once again the forefoot step is used.

After this little excursion, which, by the way, could have been extended a lot further, you will certainly agree with me when I say that you are a genuine forefoot stepper. At least some of the time. Now you're probably going to present two gait styles to me where this is precisely not the case: namely walking and jogging.

And I totally agree with you, because if it were any different, there wouldn't be any reason for me to write this book. Firstly, I would like to talk about jogging, a word that originally meant "to push slightly". Apart from the fact that a lot of people do actually land with their heels on the ground first when jogging, more recent studies prove that this running style is less efficient than a style where you touch down first on the forefoot. One such study was carried out by Professor Daniel E. Lieberman at Harvard University in the United States of America. Search for Daniel Lieberman in the Internet and you'll find several interesting videos on this subject. In his studies he essentially shows that the impact that occurs when each foot lands on the ground when running is a lot greater if you land on your heel first. It is a lot gentler if the forefoot touches the ground first, before the heel is brought down. Furthermore he found out that in other cultures where people often walk around barefoot, this more economic running style is generally preferred. Amazing, right? But basically it's nothing new.

In an interview with the German newspaper "Tagesspiegel" in 2006, the great Haile

Gebrselassie once said about his running style, which has given him so much success, "It's a matter of technique and running style. As I've said before, my style is somewhat like a ball that bounces on the ground. I don't roll my foot at all".

The legendary people of Tarahumara in Mexico, whom Christopher McDougall introduces in his bestseller "Born to Run", also accomplish an almost unbelievable running performance barefoot or in minimal shoes, also using the forefoot step pattern.

Without knowing Gebrselassie that well, it's interesting that at least Professor Liebermann, who, in his video, demonstratively jogs barefoot with a forefoot strike through the streets of New York, chooses not to implement the same concept during regular walking and even admits that he does not recognize this as a feasible concept for his life. I for one cannot help smiling at the thought of such an intelligent man who neglects to put two and two together and recognize the (in)consistency here. But sometimes it feels like the old adage with the forest that cannot be seen for the trees.

Now let's get back to walking, because that's what this book is all about. You might be asking yourself by now, how can it be that you should ideally be using the forefoot step and yet when you walk you automatically roll down from the heel. We're told from an early age on to gently "roll off" our feet when we walk (and not stomp). Global footwear-producing corporations manufacture special shoes for us so we can roll our feet better, while resourceful salesmen sell us shoes with round soles similar to those allegedly worn by the African Massai tribe. Anything to be able to roll better. Isn't it adorable how much they care? But is all that necessary? Or does it maybe help the shoe manufacturer more than us?

Perhaps we should start with a proper definition. An object that is round can roll, we can agree on that. A ball, for example, is a convex-shaped object. Such a convex shape has the ability to roll, which is quite understandable. So shoe manufacturers are not trying to adjust their shoes to such convex forms without good reason. Now let's take a look at a healthy foot. I'll try to avoid technical terms if possible because it's important for me to be understood by all. In a standing

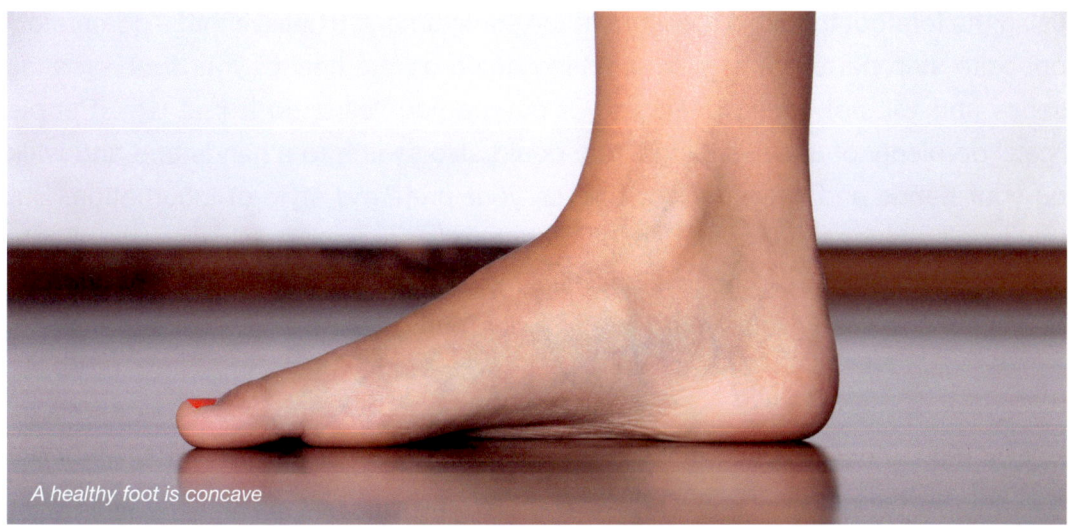
A healthy foot is concave

position, a normal foot has the forefoot, the heel and the outside edge of the sole in contact with the floor. In the center we have the so-called arch, which is not in contact with the floor. If you take a look at the foot now, you can see that it is shaped exactly opposite to the shape of a ball. It is concave! How is a concave shape supposed to roll? For comparison, you could place a soup bowl on the table with the open side facing down and wait for it to roll. To save you some time I'll tell you right now: it won't!

Really smart people will now argue: "But the heel is round". Fine and good, but what function do the arches have then? If you roll over the heel, the arch is merely rolled flat. In fact, it serves as an excellent shock absorber, as Professor Lieberman's studies also show. But only when the foot is used the way it is intended. Let us think for a moment about why shoe manufacturers (must) sell shoes with heel cushioning and well-engineered pads in the heel area. Certainly not because this style of walking is so ideal. It's interesting to know that body parts have certain anatomic functions. For example, it's better to use your knee as a knee or it could pop. By the same token, it's better to use your hand as a hand or you'll start having problems and even pain.

Now, we have established that in a number of situations you initiate movement by using the forefoot to take a step, but at the same time you believe that a completely opposite step pattern – namely touching down on the heel of your foot – makes sense and will not cause damage? Of course you "can" do it that way. People "can" do plenty of useless things. You could also switch to a handstand and walk on your hands and even declare that as your preferred style of locomotion. But that won't change the fact that neither your hands nor your shoulders were built to permanently carry your body weight this way. Unfortunately, your body is capable of adjusting to such misuse for a relatively long time before any serious damage is caused.

But by then, most of the time it's already too late. This is also the case with your foot and lower leg muscles, which are no more intended for two completely different movement concepts than your hands and shoulders are. The result of using your heels the wrong way can result in countless foot disorders ranging from heel pain to fallen arches or flatfoot.

Let's return for a moment to our tiny people, the toddlers who are just beginning to walk. The question is, if we all start off walking with a forefoot step, why do we then end up walking with a heel strike? There are various theories as to why and when humans began walking by rolling over from the heel. Dr. Greb describes one of these interpretations in his book "GODO® Mit dem Herzen gehen – Der Gang des Neuen Menschen" (walking with the heart – the walk of new-age people). This book is basically about the sedentary lifestyle of modern-day man, who feels comfortable with his "territory" and no longer has to creep through the woods in an attentive, quiet and careful way and deal with new situations on the ground. When there's no danger of stepping on a pointed twig or sharp stone and getting hurt or scaring off the targeted prey through loud trampling, one can easily get away with a sloppy rearfoot strike. Whether or not things evolved like that is something that can no longer be clarified. And at the end of the day, the "why" is quite secondary anyway.

With reference to people today, it's very likely that we learned the heel strike at around age 3, after having walked the right way – with the forefoot step – up to that point. Unlike our neighbors in the animal kingdom, we humans are strongly dependent on learning through observing. Comparative studies with bonobos and chimpanzees show that they can in some cases solve problems in their own way more quickly than human children in a similar developmental stage. Conversely, we humans are much more skilled at learning motion sequences and behavior through mimicking and, above all, sharing knowledge by passing on information, than our furry relatives. While they can acquire several different processes through observation in a lifetime, we are capable of passing on intricate processes that have been developed throughout countless lifetimes. Therefore, you can see the main reason why we fly to the moon while apes are still swinging from tree to tree. Starting around age 3, human children have the possibility to adopt walking patterns from the people around them, which they unfortunately do just as they adopt postures or gestures and facial expressions from parents or caregivers. A slouched back or a specific walk is often falsely blamed on genetics. You often hear, "Oh yes, I inherited that from my father/mother" in context with such inadequacies, when they have in fact simply copied it. Just like walking with the heel strike.

To encourage you to think about all this a bit at the end of this chapter, please follow me on a little journey:
Picture yourself on a beautiful beach. The view is fantastic, you hear the gushing of waves, feel the breeze on your skin, smell the ocean and taste the slight saltiness of the sea air on your lips. But this beautiful beach has a slight disadvantage, which you notice as you look down at your feet. This is not a sandy beach. Small, sharp fragments of seashells and pointed stones are strewn about on the ground. After enjoying the beautiful view you decide to go back to your sun lounger where you've left your shoes. You are barefoot. You carefully take your first step towards your chair – now how did you just place your foot on the ground?

I'm very sure you just placed the ball of your foot onto the ground really carefully. See, when we move across rough and unknown terrain with unshod feet, we automatically switch to the forefoot step. Just like in various other areas, when necessary our brains switch over to the behavior and movement patterns of our ancestors, which were accepted for thousands of years. The same applies here too. Stepping on a stone or a pointed stick with your heel is just too big a risk. Try it for yourself. And while doing so think about evolution, God, Allah or whoever created you barefoot. Every cell of our bodies has been adjusting to this type of movement for thousands of years. Do you still have any doubts as to what your natural style of locomotion is?

The "hearing test"

Don't worry, this chapter isn't about me finding out how often you take your Walkman or mp3 player with you on walks or how often you go to rock concerts. I merely wish to demonstrate to you one more time the difference between the two walking patterns you have at your disposal, and to this end I invite you to take a little test:

Please take off your shoes so you are either barefoot or only wearing socks. Hold your ears closed. Use your index fingers to completely shut your ear canals. Now take a couple of steps the way you are used to walking.

You are probably hearing a muffled "boom-boom" sound. Take a couple more steps and actively listen to this sound. Every step you take compresses your joints so the shock waves travel along your spine up to your skull where you experience the "boom-boom". Every one of your steps is therefore sending little shockwaves throughout your whole body, which naturally strains your joints and leads to dete-

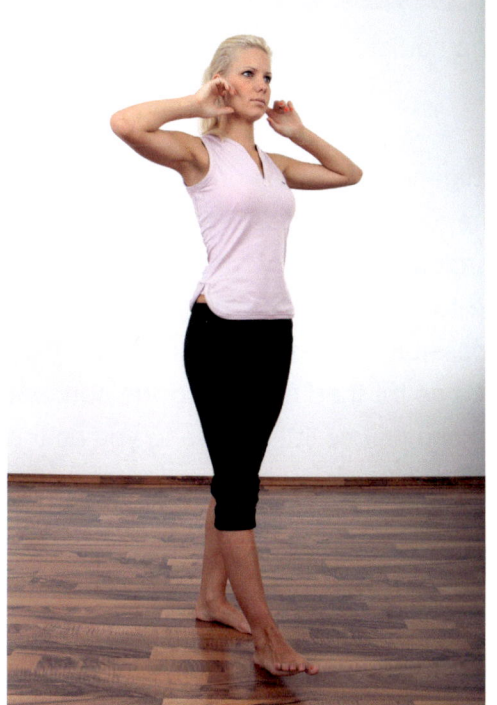

rioration. Just think about how many steps you take in a day. How many in a year? And throughout your lifetime?

Well, that is the rearfoot step or heel strike!

Take a short break.

Now hold your ears closed again. Take a couple of steps and instead of your heel, try placing the ball of your foot on the ground first and then letting your heel follow. You might remember sneaking around playing "Indian" as a child and how you tip-toed around on the balls of your feet. Try switching between these gait patterns and you'll notice that you can't hear a sound during the forefoot step and therefore no shock waves are being sent through your body either.

Essentially, that is the principle of the forefoot step!

Perplexing, isn't it? This little test is a simple and yet impressive method of pointing out the difference between the forefoot and the heel step. I've been using it for years and have my clients do it, and they are often amazed and aghast at the same time about how crude and noisy their normal movement pattern is, in comparison to the forefoot step. I think you might almost be convinced and we can begin with the first preliminary exercise. Should you live in an

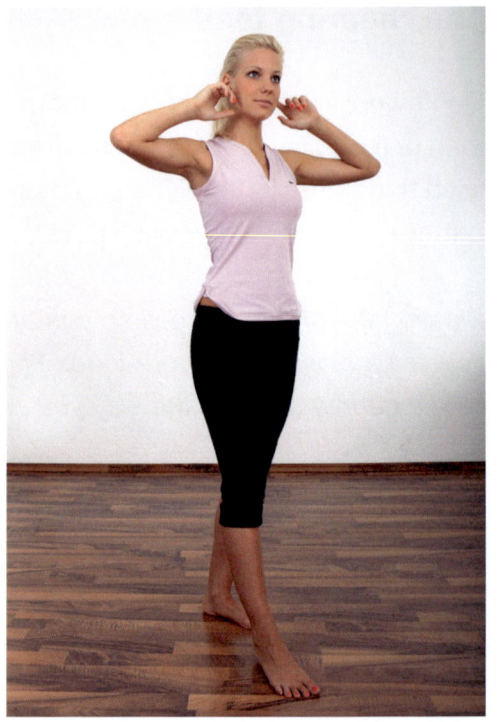

apartment with tenants living above you, you can quickly find out which movement patterns your neighbors are using. Just listen.

Speaking of which, of course there are still indigenous peoples on our planet who enjoy a more simple life and move through the forest and steppes using only the forefoot step. You may be surprised to know that our concept of "growing tired from running/walking" is normally incomprehensible to these people. They simply can't grasp it and their language doesn't make it possible to describe it in a way they would understand either. Perplexing, isn't it? It's as if I tried explaining the concept of "relaxation through stress" to you. It would make just as little sense to you as the fact that someone could grow tired from running or walking makes to these people.

Getting to know your feet

Since, like most people, you probably know your feet by sight rather than knowing them as the wonderful tools for touching and feeling that they are, I would like to invite you to partake in a little preliminary exercise in order to restore contact.

In the 1960s there was a disaster in the pharmaceutical world that came to be known as the Contergan scandal. Contergan was a new drug that was prescribed to pregnant women for nausea and its side effects led to deformed arms in many babies. Or you may have seen people before who have lost their arms in an accident. What I'm trying to say is this: a disability in one area very often leads to a much higher ability in another one.

People who cannot use their arms have often learned to use their legs for many tasks that you and I would carry out with our arms. These people succeed in drawing or writing with their feet and master many other everyday activities as well.

In 2010, 23-year-old pianist Liu Wei won the Chinese equivalent of the TV casting show "Got Talent". The special thing about this is that when he was 10 years old Liu Wei lost both of his arms by accidentally touching a high-voltage cable when he was playing with his friends. He later defied fate and learned to play the piano with his toes.

The interesting thing about this story is that you'd probably have trouble just moving one toe if I asked you to, even though Liu Wei has the same muscles, bones, fascia, arteries and veins in his legs and feet as you and I. It's somewhat intimidating when you're struggling to wiggle your little toe while your neighbor is able to recite a piece from Mozart. But not to worry, you don't have to.

These examples are only intended to show you what possibilities are out there. Your body is in fact aligned in such a way that your arms are made for mobility while your legs are in charge of stability. And yet this stability requires a certain amount of flexibility in order to prevent injuries and to be able to act dynamically. But enough said: Let's begin the preliminary exercise.

(1) Please take off your shoes. Stand relaxed and straight, either barefoot or in stocking feet. Now imagine a thread attached to the top of your head, gently pulling you upwards like a puppet. Your body remains completely relaxed. Your head rises with ease, but without your neck muscles tensing up. You let your gaze wander horizontally. You might feel as though you are making a slight double chin. Good. Keep your jaw muscles relaxed too. Your lips may slightly part.

Your arms are dangling relaxed at your sides. Feel the weight of your arms and let them be pulled down by gravity. Relax your stomach and buttocks and make sure that your knees are slightly bent and not stretched. From now on we shall call this pose the "neutral position".

Feel into your body. Take note of the position of your head, whether one shoulder is hanging lower than the other, perhaps because you're holding one shoulder up higher without meaning to. Can you manage to relax your stomach and pelvis and just "let go"? How is your pelvis positioned in your body and which leg are you putting more weight on? Are you standing on your entire foot or rather on the ball of your foot or your heel? Is your foot buckling over the inner side more or is your weight on the outer side? Take note.

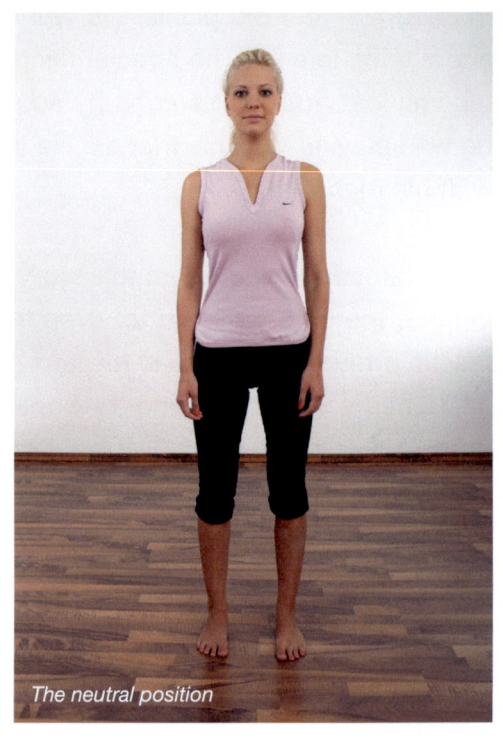

The neutral position

(2) Relax. Now slowly shift your weight to the balls of your feet and take note of what happens. How are the muscles in your feet reacting? What are your leg muscles doing and how is the rest of your body reacting? Begin to slowly shift your weight onto your heels. Feel the difference in your body and in your feet. Take your time and slowly shift your weight back and forth a

couple of times. Take a couple of seconds to slowly transfer the weight from your heels to the balls of your feet.

Once you think you've gotten the idea and wish to move on to the next step, just take it. But first, stand relaxed in the neutral position and linger a moment to appreciate the changes in your body.

(3) Now very slowly transfer your weight onto the outer side of your right foot and the inner side of your left foot. How are the muscles in your feet reacting and what are the muscles in your lower leg doing? How are your pelvis and your upper body adjusting? Now roll your weight onto the other side, again really slowly: Left foot – outer side, right foot – inner side. Good. Make note of the differences between these sides. Take your time to shift your weight a couple of times. Here too, you should closely monitor what happens when you switch from one side to the other. Take your time so you have the chance to experience the changes.

Once you think you've gotten the idea and wish to move on to the next step, just take it. But first, stand relaxed in the neutral position and linger a moment to appreciate the changes in your body.

(4)) Imagine your feet standing on the face of a clock. It's 12 o'clock in front of you and 6 o'clock behind you. The dial is divided into hours and minutes. Surely you know the difference between high-quality clocks and cheap ones. While the second hand of cheap clocks often "skips" a second, the hands of high-quality clocks usually glide evenly from one second to the next. I would like you to glide around the face of the clock like the second hand of a high-quality clock. Begin by transferring your weight onto the balls of your feet – on to 12 o'clock. From here you shift your weight slowly towards 3 o'clock – by putting weight on the outer side of your right foot and the inner side of your left one. Slowly move around this imaginary clock in a circular motion. From here you slowly move on towards 6 o'clock – weight on your heels – and then in a wide curve past 9 o'clock – outer side left, inner side right – and back up to 12 o'clock. Take note of the feeling in your feet. What are your legs doing, your pelvis, your upper body? Take your time to step

around the face of the clock a couple of times.

Do this exercise as slowly as possible. And don't worry: it's normal to have trouble balancing at first. At the same time you're training your sense of balance, as a small side effect. Move clockwise first and then counter-clockwise. Briefly pause before changing directions and feel and observe to what extent you experience one direction differently than the other.

A variation of this exercise is to pivot in 15-minute intervals. For example, from 12 to 3 and back to 12. Or from 9 to 6 and back to 9. This slightly smaller set of movements provides a good "in-between" exercise, which you can do on the fly at a bus stop or waiting in line at the cinema.

Once you've practiced these very easy preliminary exercises slowly and consciously for a while, you'll notice several positive effects. Without going into too much detail, it can be said that muscle tension and tissue adhesions in the foot and lower leg area will subside considerably after a while. These structural issues arise after decades of incorrect weight-bearing through using the heel strike. Results include immobile foot and ankle areas that are prone to sprains and "twisting". Another benefit of this exercise is an improved perception of your feet and, of course, better balance. Practicing the neutral position also leads to better overall body perception and – if you take your time and consciously work on it – a decline in tension in the entire musculature. If you like, you can compare it to complete relaxation. Similar effects have been reached through numerous forms of meditation or chi-gong exercises for thousands of years. However, they are usually more complicated and shrouded in mystery. Sometimes it works very simply without all the "chi" and "chakras", which are nothing but tools from my point of view. But if these work for you, go ahead and use them. Otherwise you can happily leave the "chi" to the "Chi-nese".

The forefoot step

The forefoot step, or natural step as I like to call it, has many benefits when compared to the heel step. It's very easy, but at the same time very complex. After many, many years of working with numerous clients I have noticed that it's often too complex to grasp immediately. There are many fine details that must be considered and, if you try to focus on all of these at once, chances are that you'll quickly become frustrated by something that is supposed to be fun and you may even put the "forefoot step" quickly aside again, because you think you have better things to do. That would be a shame, because the benefits of the forefoot step may not always be recognizable at the very beginning. "Haste makes waste", as the old saying goes. Walking or running are processes that are for the most part internalized actions. You've been set on autopilot so to speak and all you have to do is enter your destination. Patients in rehabilitation become painfully aware of how complex and demanding the process of "walking" is when they are faced with the difficult task of having to relearn this process after an accident – and they are usually taught wrong all over again. But patients in rehabilitation don't have much of a choice, do they? They either learn to walk or they don't walk, and that clearly makes the effort worthwhile.

However, you are now in a different the situation: You already have a functioning gait pattern, even if it isn't the most efficient one. And now I am asking you for nothing less than to replace your working pattern with another one in mid-step, so to speak. In the computer world, replacing a working system while the computer is still running is extremely risky and deeply troubles IT specialists. It is easier to erase the existing system and install a new one. That is the situation in which patients in rehabilitation find themselves. However, I am more than certain that staying at such a clinic for several months is not really an option for you. So we must adjust and change the system while it's still running.

But first things first. Before I am able to successfully reconfigure your walk to the forefoot mode, I will first need a couple of things from you.

Time:

Please note that it will certainly take a while until you have completely changed your gait pattern. At the beginning you will have to do the forefoot step quite intentionally. As soon as you go back on autopilot, you'll probably fall back into the old pattern. It will take some time until you feel confident enough with the new gait pattern and your nervous system is able to compare both patterns and select the forefoot step automatically.

Play instinct:

When approaching the following exercises or the preliminary exercises, you should enjoy what you are doing, which is the best prerequisite for learning something new. Do the exercises whenever you feel like it; if you don't feel like it once in a while just skip your "training". Simply enjoy discovering and experimenting. You can safely feel that you've learned something and are making progress when you do something the wrong way and notice it yourself. Forget about frustration and stress. It is your pace, your learning curve and your results. Have fun with it!

Slowing down:

If you perform the exercises very slowly, it will benefit your perception and your learning progress. I always tell my clients: "As slowly as possible without having to stop or interrupt your movement." This way you will succeed in truly reintegrating the whole process of movement without skipping any part of the process. You will note that it's immensely more difficult to do something very slowly than to do the same thing quickly. If you are able to perform a movement in slow motion, you'll also be able to do it faster. The other way around is a different story. Many people can't even keep their balance when walking very slowly, even though they walk around at a normal speed several hours a day.

Imagination:

This refers to the technique of visualizing things. In general, it doesn't make such a big difference to your brain whether you actually perform an activity or just vividly imagine performing it. The same areas of the brain are active. This is the reason why athletes, for instance, employ visualization techniques to enhance their performance. When in bed, riding a train or on a plane, all you have to do is visualize how to do the forefoot step. Imagine what it feels like, what it looks like, what it sounds like and be as specific and detailed as possible. This way you can train the forefoot step mentally, even if you aren't yet able to do it physically.

The next section describes what to do with your body.
In my practice, it has been a tried and proven technique to instruct clients in the forefoot step in three phases. The sequence in which you perform the exercises is left completely up to you.
1. How do I use my feet?
2. How do I use my arms?
3. What moves me forward?

1. How do I use my feet?
Since you've already become acquainted with your feet during the introductory phase, you will now learn what your feet are actually doing in the forefoot step. First assume the neutral position, with which you've already familiarized yourself. Please take off your shoes for this purpose. And here we go:

(1) Starting in the neutral position shift your weight on to one leg, the supporting leg, (in this example we start with the left leg) until you have the impression that there is no weight at all on the other one (in our example the right leg), the free leg. Then let your pelvis glide slightly back into your body by further relaxing your stomach. Now let your free leg, the right one, slowly swing forward. Your whole leg should be completely relaxed. It's like having a small string attached to your knee, which is lifting your leg slightly and moving it forward. You will note how your pelvis is involved in this forward motion.

(2) Your right foot should be completely relaxed, hanging down at a slight angle. It's the same sensation that you have when sitting on a wall and letting your feet swing freely. (This is the key element of the exercise.)

(3) Now let your foot touch the floor in its relaxed state. If you have done it well, you will notice that your foot touches the ground first with the ball on the right side, then with the ball on the inside and only at the end with the heel.

(4) Slowly apply weight on the right foot and let the left foot slowly swing forward. Follow steps (1) to (3) with your left foot and take a couple of steps.

Make sure that you perform this exercise slowly, focusing on each step.

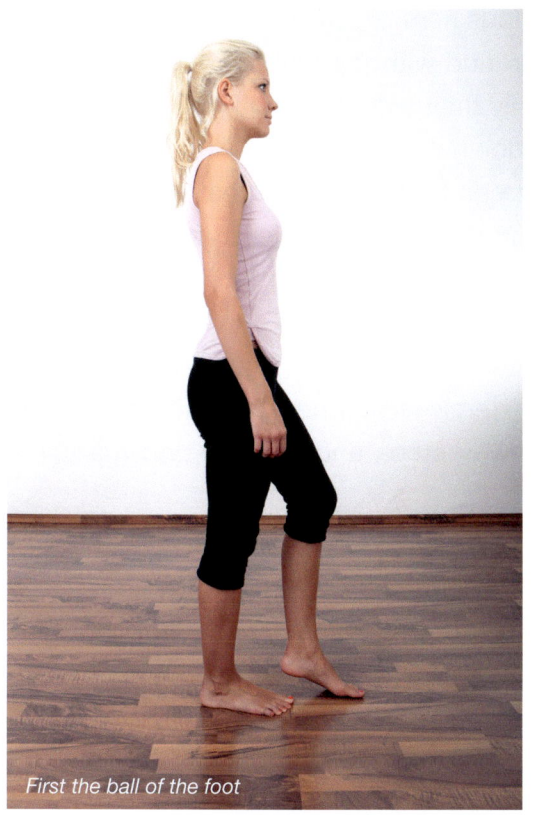

First the ball of the foot

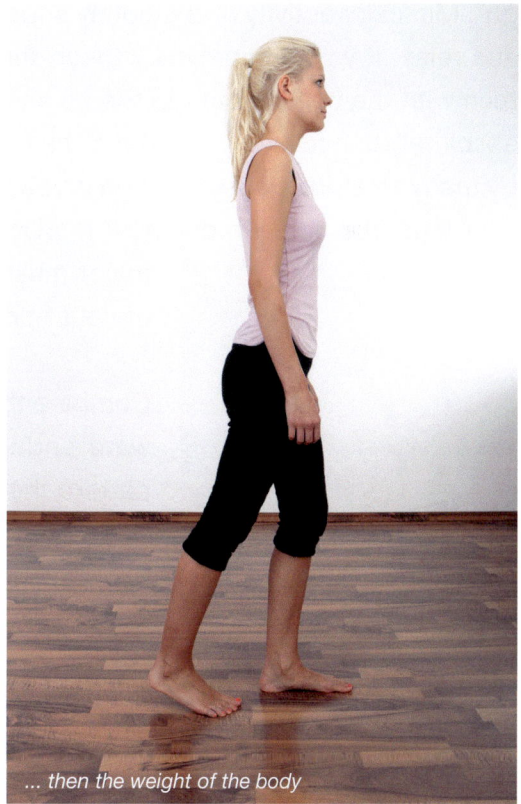

... then the weight of the body

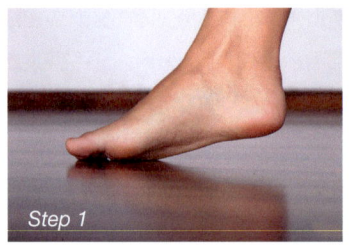
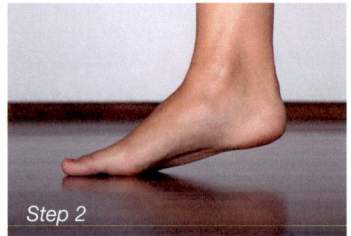
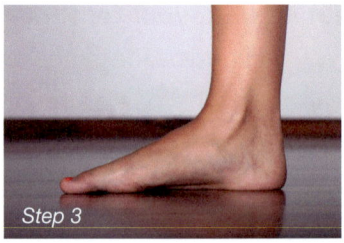

Step 1   Step 2   Step 3

Take several small steps and let each foot touch the ground naturally. Always keep your torso straight and your stomach relaxed. Don't look down at your feet, but rather straight ahead.

So now you know exactly how the ball of the foot touches the ground with the forefoot step. The key is to leave the foot completely relaxed in the ankle. Through decades of walking and running from heel to toe you have developed the habit of pulling your toes and your foot up with your muscles. You must learn again to "let go". Muscular activity is absolutely superfluous here. If you let your foot hang down and relax, it will automatically touch the ground with the ball of your little toe (1), then with the ball of your big toe (2) and only then with the heel (3). Therefore, it is absolutely unnecessary to extend the foot downward, as is often wrongly assumed by many forefoot steppers. Even if you've been told in the past that you should lift your legs, the actual movement is made by the flexor muscle of your hip (psoas major muscle). Simply move your leg from the center of your body.

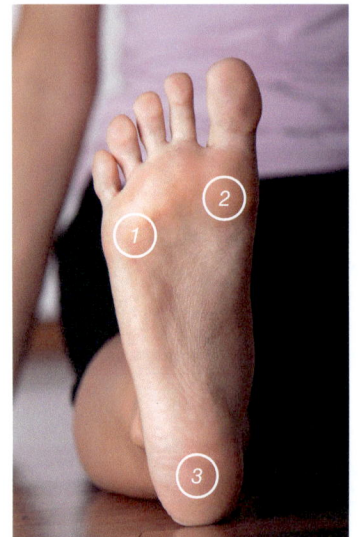

Combine this exercise every now and then with backward and sideway steps and you will find the same pattern there.

Experiment with this exercise whenever you feel like it. Take 5 minutes to observe closely and to work slowly. Don't worry if you have difficulties integrating this exercise into your daily activities at first. Wearing shoes with heels and having other things on your mind will make it harder for you to learn a new movement pattern. This is completely normal. In stressful situations your brain will fall back on tried and proven gait patterns, even though those might not be ideal.

You'll need a little time and a few quiet moments to familiarize your control center with the forefoot step again and get accustomed to it, which will probably happen sooner than you think. After all, as you are now aware, you used to know this style of walking when you were little!

2. How do I use my arms?

"What do you actually do with your arms when you walk?" Every time I ask my clients this, they reach unexpected heights of creativity. The arms should swing, they should be left relaxed and still, the forearm moves or the whole arm and "sometimes one way, sometimes another" – these are just a few of the answers I hear every day.

For one, holding the arms relaxed and motionless next to your body is completely wrong and absolute nonsense. This can already be seen in how this instruction is worded. "Relaxed" and actively "holding the arms" is a contradiction in terms. Some people falsely assume that their arms are relaxed when they're slouching with their hands in the pockets of their trousers or jackets. The explanation for this takes us back several thousand years in the history of our evolution.

Our ancestors originally moved on all fours and then gradually (or rather step by step) developed the upright walk. Even though we no longer really use our arms when walking, generally speaking we still maintain the movement pattern of walking on all fours. The arms and legs on each side move in opposite directions. By the way, this is also true for our relatives in the trees. Among experts this is known as "contralateral movement". Except for the first step, where the arm and leg move on the same side in the same direction, the left arm and the right leg or the right arm and the left leg alternately move forward. This movement pattern is what stabilizes your gait. You'll notice this in particular when you start to run. Try to run really fast and then move the same arm and the leg on the same side forward. You won't be able to do it.

Now try walking with your hands in your pockets, or holding on to a purse or hand-bag or simply try "holding your arms relaxed at your sides"; to do so, you will have to suppress this contralateral movement by tensing up your muscles. Holding your arms still requires more strength than letting them swing loosely and naturally back and forth. In fact, it's not the arms and legs that move in opposite directions, but rather the pelvis and the shoulder girdle. Your arms naturally follow the movements of the shoulder girdle without any tension, just like your legs follow the movements of your pelvis. This way, all your movements originate from the center of your body and are much more efficient.

Another thing I've learned while working with my clients is that many people move their arms, but leave the shoulder girdle motionless. Again a movement is sup-pressed and held back here. As you know, the pelvis and shoulder girdle are con-nected by the spine. Normally, the spine twists like a spiral in one or the other direction with every step you take. But when you hold your shoulder girdle still, this movement is suppressed. It's an interesting observation that people who move this way are more restricted in their mobility and suffer from pain in the very same area. This hardly comes as a surprise, since the muscle must be permanently tense in order to suppress a natural movement. I think now you've got the concept, so let's move on to the exercise.

First assume the neutral position, with which you have already become familiar. And here we go:

(1) To start with, take a couple of steps in your usual gait pattern. If you haven't yet internalized placing the ball of your foot first on the floor, feel free to use the pattern you use every day. We need you to focus on something else here.
(2) Observe your shoulder girdle and your pelvis. Do you feel the contralateral movement? What are your arms doing? What about your spine? First observe.

You don't have to change anything for now. The point is to realize how you walk.

(3) Stop for a moment. Let your arms hang down relaxed at your sides. Imagine that your arms are in the sleeves of a heavy, wet coat. Your arms are completely relaxed. Slightly elevate your head as if it were filled with helium. Now start walking again and observe how these changes influence your gait.

(4) As your arms swing lightly and relaxed at the sides of your body, pay full attention to the contralateral movements of your pelvis and shoulder girdle. Can you recognize the contralateral movement? What happens when you let it gradually increase? Play a little with this movement and slowly find the point where you notice the greatest possible contralateral movement. How do these changes influence the movements of your relaxed arms? Observe and perceive. Exaggerate the movements, if you like, and make them as big as possible. In any case, observe that pelvis and shoulder girdle move contralaterally.

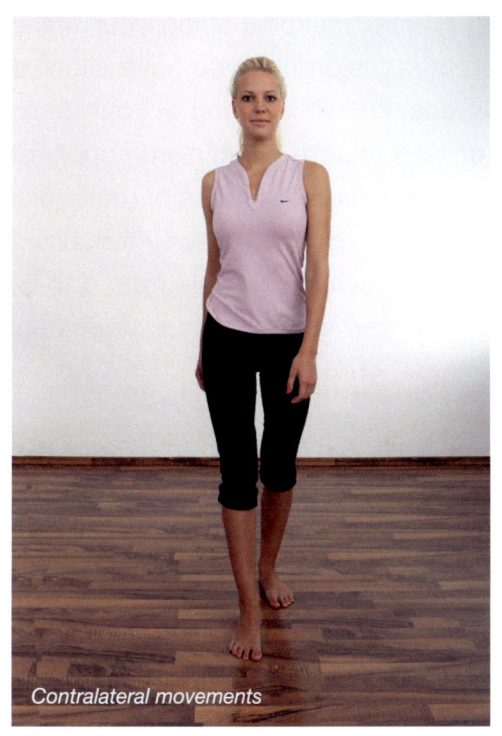
Contralateral movements

(5) Now decrease the size of the contralateral movements. Find a level that is comfortable for you without letting the movements disappear completely. Stop focusing now on your shoulders and your pelvis. Observe how your spine slightly rotates with each step. Let the contralateral movement originate now from the center of your body by allowing your spine to participate in the contralateral movements. Notice how your movement pattern changes and how fluently and elegantly your arms move in harmony with your body. Focus on this new gait for several minutes.

(6) If you still remember your gait pattern during step (1), then use it now, alternating

several times between your old and your new gait pattern and compare. What differences do you notice?

As always do this exercise slowly, being aware of each step, and focus on your observations. As with the other exercises, the "wrongs" you notice are very important for you, because realizing how something doesn't work is the first step towards learning something new.

This exercise can be easily integrated into your everyday activities. Even if placing the forefoot first on the ground requires a lot of attention in the beginning, you can also train your body's contralateral movements using the incorrect heel step. Do this exercise consciously, whenever you feel like it. No matter if at home, on your way to work or while shopping, the whole world is your gym!

And I have another tip for you: If you have an office job and often suffer from back pain after a long day of work, this exercise is just right for you. The contralateral movements and activation of the smaller and greater muscles along your spine that help to twist it with every step will loosen the tension that you have allowed to build up by "holding" your body in a certain position while sitting at your desk. The slight movements will help to relax tension and restore a sufficient supply of blood and nutrients to the affected areas, while promoting elimination of metabolic waste products. At the same time this also means that once you have internalized the forefoot step, you'll automatically do this exercise when you walk from A to B. Any back pain will take care of itself and you'll no longer have to do any additional exercises.

3. What moves me forward?

Many people ask themselves this question with regard to their careers or athletic capabilities. What moves me forward in my job? How can I make progress on my athletic proficiency scale? Of course, this is a valid question in these areas of your life, but I'd like you to put this question on a much more elementary level: What moves me forward when I walk?

During a stroll through the park or walking around town you can easily get the impression that there must be more than one answer to this question, especially when you pay attention to the people around you. One guy shuffles his feet forward, dutifully dragging the rest of his body behind. Another seems to be pulled forward by an invisible thread that is attached to her head, almost as if her head were leading the rest of her body by a neck's length and dominating the entire walking process. Then there are some who push their pelvis forward. But we could go on like this forever. In most cases the way these folks walk is the result of a specific posture typical for them. Just observe the people around you and you'll understand what I mean.

So what is the correct way to walk? There is a great phrase which I believe was coined by the famous manual therapist Dr. Ida Rolf: "Walking is a matter of falling and catching yourself." But what does that mean?

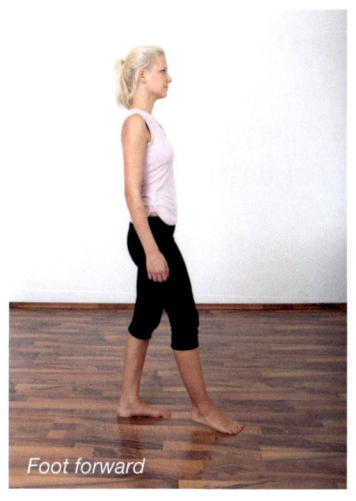
Foot forward

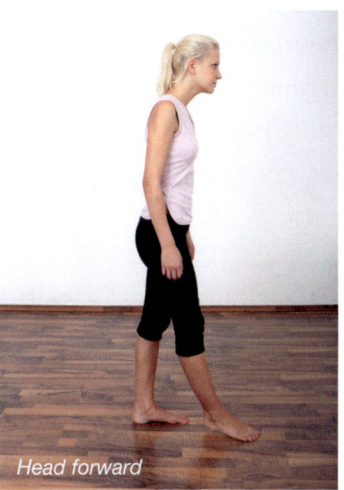
Head forward

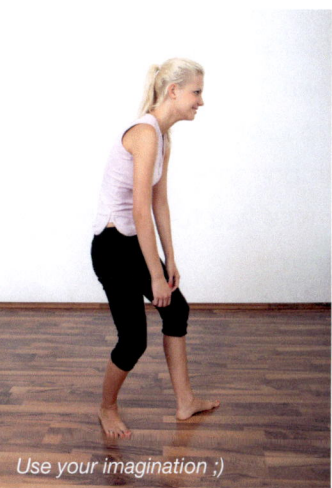
Use your imagination ;)

Here again we can learn from children who are just learning to walk. These little people stand as straight as a board. Once they've decided where they want to go, they lean forward until they nearly lose their balance and off they go. The feet follow the momentum of the body in small steps (on the forefoot) and our toddler is up and running. If they are still a little shaky on the legs and lose their balance, they end up on their bellies completely relaxed. This can startle them briefly and make them cry, but usually nothing happens, as the child's body is too relaxed to be hurt. In this context I wouldn't advise you to land on your belly like a toddler, because the average adult is so tense that the result might be a knocked-out tooth or broken hand. Just one more thing you were able to do better in the past. But let's get back to walking.

Just as with our novice walkers, most adults move with a certain level of function-ality when they want to go faster. When you sprint you usually push your torso forward. This gives your body weight a forward momentum, which you only need to push a little. Very few people would ever consider leaning backward when run-ning to catch a bus. Reduce the speed, however, and you get what most people do when they walk. Contrary to what we used to do during the first days of our "walking careers", we no longer make use of gravity and our body weight to get moving. We could philosophize almost endlessly about the reason for this here. There are entire fields of body therapy which deal with attributing certain psycholo-gical properties to your gait and which will label you based on the way you walk. Of course, there is some truth to what they say. But I've learned that instead of asking "why" it's the "how" that is significantly more interesting and productive. How do you actually walk? What would it be like if you walked in a different way? And most importantly: What possibilities could it open up for you? For further elaboration, I invite you to take this little test:

For a moment forget everything you've learned so far in this book about the fore-foot step and functional walking. Just remember how you used to walk before you read this book. Now take a few steps across the room and observe from which body part your movement originates. Try to find the engine of your movement. What pulls or pushes you forward and what dictates your direction? Be honest with yourself. This is not about doing it right or wrong. I promise you that I won't suddenly appear from between the pages of this book and loudly shout, "You're doing it all wrong!" Finding out how you do something, even though it's wrong, is a first enormous step towards improvement. Take a few steps and observe.

Since you are now reading this line, I assume that you've finished your exercise and are ready for the next step. The result you got is actually quite inconsequential at this point. Maybe it was your head, your feet, your pelvis or some other body part that pushed or pulled you. Remember your movement pattern so that you can compare it to the method I'm about to introduce to you.

(1) Take up the neutral position.

(2) Very slowly shift your weight forward. Leave both feet on the ground until you're about to lose your balance and have to take a step to avoid landing face down on the floor. As soon as you have the feeling that taking a step is inevitable, just go with the flow.

(3) Keep the forward tilt of your body so that you have to take another step, and another one, and another one.

I have to admit that you'll probably be stumbling forward in a rather uncoordinated fashion at this point. And of course you shouldn't walk down the street like that. I'd hate to see you get arrested for disorderly conduct! But anyway, if you did the exercise right, you must have noticed something. Even though I didn't tell you to go faster, you probably noticed that you gained momentum with each step and even though you were going pretty fast, you didn't use much energy. You were more relaxed than you were strained. In this case you let gravity work for you. That's what I call efficiency.

You can transfer this phenomenon to your regular walking style with ease. Imagine that someone had attached a thread to your torso at the level of the solar plexus.

With every step you take, your body is gently pulled forward by this thread. At the level of the solar plexus, pinch your shirt or sweater between your thumb and index finger and tug on it, pulling your body forward. Your legs will automatically follow your body and walking suddenly becomes quite an easy thing to do. Of course, you don't have to constantly pull at your clothes in everyday life. It will suffice to slowly shift your balance forward a little and let the rest just happen.

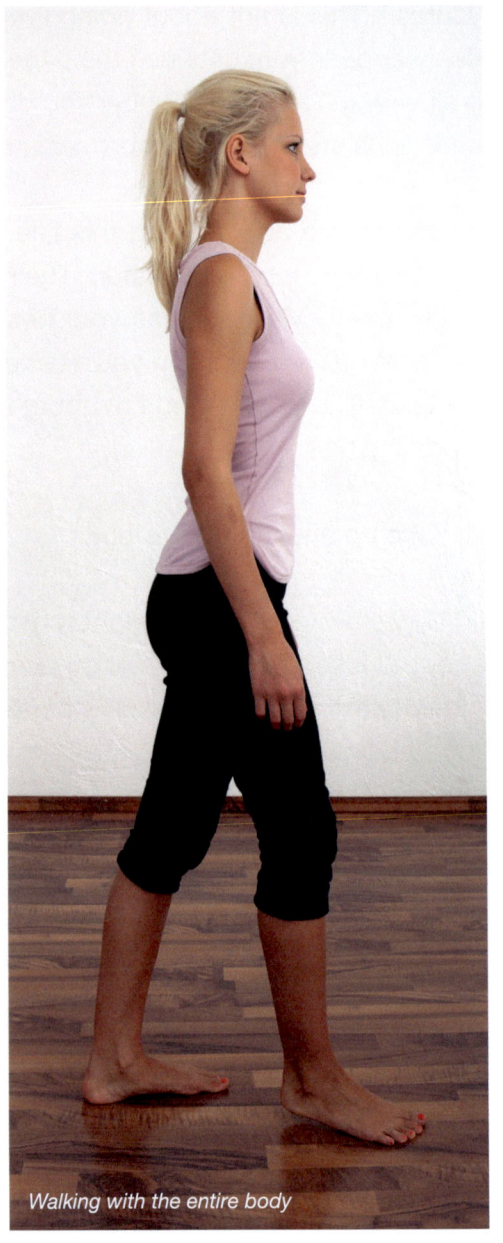

Walking with the entire body

Finale

This is where we come around full-circle. You now have all the elements of the functional forefoot step in front of you and all you need to do is put them together. But before you do, I'd like to point out a couple of important aspects that you might have already noticed yourself.

Many trainers of the forefoot step only focus on the feet and forget to point out this issue, but when you move forward simply with the help of gravity, you'll note that it is suddenly much easier to place the forefoot on the ground first. And if you stay relaxed, your shoulder girdle and your pelvis will suddenly make contralateral movements and your arms will gently swing back and forth by themselves. These three simple exercises result in the functional forefoot step. Even though every part is relatively easy in itself, it is difficult to handle all three simultaneously. Which is why I intentionally deal with each one separately.

As soon as you feel comfortable with the individual exercises, you can start to combine them. When you succeed in combining all three areas, then you can train the forefoot step at any time and wherever you are. Special exercises or training units will no longer be necessary. Later on, you can simply stop using them altogether. Every day and every step will then be a training unit for you and you'll be surprised at how fast you make progress.

Voilà! Now you've got it: the forefoot step! That's all you need to know. That's all you need to be capable of doing. But it never hurts to know a bit more.

The right speed counts

Before we turn to the question of footwear, I'd like to point out one more important thing to you. There is one question I've been frequently asked for years, by clients who have just learned the forefoot step from me: "Why is it so difficult to implement it in everyday life?"

Many of my clients say that they think the forefoot step is a wonderful thing and also implement it regularly at home. Many have also been happily jogging or hiking across the globe for years using the forefoot step. But at the office, when shopping or in other everyday situations they often find it difficult and return to their old pattern. Why is that?

The cause lies in two very essential factors. One of them is the right footwear. You will find all you need to know about that in the next chapter. High heels and toes wedged into narrow shoes will make walking with the forefoot step virtually impossible. The second factor is the speed at which you walk.

Walking briskly often dominates everyday life for many people. In other words, they don't stride slowly and neither do they trot, but rather choose a speed somewhere in between. A "fast walk" so to speak. It is the speed at which you walk when you're in a hurry, either because you want to catch the next train, have an appointment or simply have no time. Quite interestingly, the forefoot step doesn't work right, or at least not perfectly, at this speed. So I wonder, of course, why this particular speed makes it difficult to perform the forefoot step. Here is my conclusion: because this speed doesn't really exist!

Why should this speed not exist, I hear you ask. Didn't Mr. Beckmann explain it so aptly a few sentences ago? Of course it exists! It's just not inherent in nature. When you move slowly, you take slow steps and the forefoot step works just fine. You can speed up to the point where you would normally get to your "fast walk". However, you should actually start to slightly trot at this point, a type of movement you can perform easily with the forefoot step. You can effortlessly implement the forefoot step in anything from a slower gait to a fast run. So in my opinion, the "fast walk" is not a natural movement pattern. When we want to get from A to B fast, we run. Normally!

But in our society running is often not considered appropriate. A client of mine, a surgeon to be more specific, once told me when I explained my thesis to him: "You know, Mr. Beckmann, that actually sounds quite reasonable. I have only one problem with it. As a doctor I'm not supposed to run to an emergency at the hospital. It would scare the patients who saw me, or at least worry them, since they'd assume that something bad had happened. That is why we got the directive from hospital management to walk briskly and not run in such a case. It attracts less attention." And this was when it hit me, because most people have their own personal "hospital management" that also tells them: "You cannot be running here and now! What kind of impression would you make? What should people think?"

So the only movement pattern where the forefoot step hardly works or only with limitations is therefore a socially constructed set of rules made by humans! Many indigenous peoples would probably be surprised by how we race around in such a hectic and uptight manner with our sharp militaristic goose-step over the heel. They'd likely wonder why we don't run if we're in such a damn hurry.

You are certainly "able" to walk very fast, but remember this: It doesn't mean that it's a functional way of walking just because we "can" do it. We can also walk on our hands or stick our imbalanced heads out in front of us. We can make all kinds of decisions that won't necessarily be good for our bodies. *How could you otherwise explain why we enjoy sports where injuries, even complicated fractures, frequently occur and why we pursue such sports anyway, sometimes even after sustaining such injuries?*

Footwear

Buying shoes is all about making decisions. Of course you can decide to wear shoes with heels or even high heels. But is that sensible? Now, to wind things up, let's have a look at this topic.

You have now familiarized yourself with the forefoot step in a short and easy way. You have analyzed your own (and by now hopefully "former") gait pattern and gra-dually replaced it with a more functional way of walking. Now, as a forefoot stepper you will also have to deal with the perennial subject of footwear in order to be happy in today's modern world. We must be honest here: Very few of us are brave enough to run around barefoot in urban Western Europe, the USA or elsewhere. But don't get me wrong! Of course it's possible and there are people who do go barefoot through our modern world in both summer and winter. That is wonderful, but in any case you must consider the possibility that your boss (should you have one) will have something to say about it at work, which will make your dreams of strutting around with unshod feet remain unfulfilled. Depending on your lifestyle, you might experience situations where people will suggest that you wear shoes. That is absolutely okay. Mind you, I wear shoes myself. But which footwear is it going to be?

It would certainly exceed the limits of this book to discuss the advantages and dis-advantages of individual shoe models in detail. All the manufacturers whose shoes have found their way into my shoe cupboard have their pros and cons. In the end personal taste also plays a significant role. But, having said that, there are some very objective criteria, which I would like to give you as a kind of guide to your next shoe-shopping spree.

Flat shoes

Simply put: your foot does not have a raised heel. So why should your shoe have one? When buying your footwear, make sure that your shoe is as flat as possible. In fact, you will probably only find very few manufacturers who offer a truly flat shoe. There are some manufacturers who explicitly advertise their shoes as being flat, but they're not. For one, the shoe sole is often not really flat, but merely has a very low heel. This effect is often intensified by putting insoles into the shoes, which creates a padded heel. These manufacturers are obviously thinking of rearfoot strikers, who need heel pads.

But heeled shoes are actually detrimental to your posture and physical structure and can often lead to various postural deformities and also painful symptoms in the back and neck. Furthermore, walking with a functional forefoot step is difficult or even impossible when wearing heeled shoes, depending on the height of the heel. So forget shoes with raised heels and go for the flats. The heel and the ball of your foot should be on the same level.

A small consolation for the ladies. Of course you won't go straight to hell for wearing high heels with your dress once in a while on a festive occasion. More importantly, you should keep an eye on what type of shoes you wear on a day-to-day basis. Your most predominant gait pattern will have the greatest impact on your body and you should be aware of the consequences. If you are really honest with yourself, whether or not you have shapely legs has more to do with your eating habits or your lifestyle and less with the shoes you wear.

Toe space
From the visual perspective, this is a rather delicate matter since we have been conditioned by shoe designers, who torture our feet on behalf of the shoe industry, to prefer shoes with pointed toes or at least a narrow shape. Of course it's interesting to keep in mind that while designers may be experts when it comes to design, they have no idea about anatomy or functional movement. Which is why our feet, especially our toes, are pushed and squeezed into the shape the designer has envisioned for us. The effects are dramatic. The hallux valgus deformity, also called bunion, is a malposition of the big toe which afflicts many people in old age. It has been verified that such foot problems are associated with wearing wrong footwear

for many years. When looking at such a person's foot, the shape is congruent to the layout of common footwear. A healthy "normal foot", which is surprisingly also a condition known to academic medicine, looks completely different.

The toes are normally slightly splayed away from each other and the big toe points straight ahead. It is absolutely essential to offer enough toe space to maintain a healthy foot. Toe space means that your toes have enough freedom to stretch out and move around. Toe space is also important for the forefoot step, because every time you place the ball of your foot on the ground your toes fan out slightly and need their space. This obviously won't work if there is no space. The forefoot step is therefore difficult and often uncomfortable in tight shoes without sufficient toe space.

This issue is especially delicate because shoes with sufficient toe space must have a more voluminous cut to provide it. Whether you become an immediate fan or need a little time to get yourself accustomed to this new style will depend on your personal taste in shoes. However, the fact of the matter is that you will definitely not want to go without your toe space, once you have grown accustomed to it.

Unfortunately, there is only a very small number of manufacturers who recognize that there is a market for such shoes. Most follow the mainstream here, thus inadvertently helping to systematically cripple your feet.

Weight

Shoes should provide conditions as close to being barefoot as possible. For this reason, they should naturally be as lightweight as possible. The weight of shoes largely depends on the thickness of the sole. This means that weight is, in a sense, an indicator for two criteria at the same time. The shoe should be light and the sole as flexible as possible. This combination usually makes for a lightweight shoe. You will probably find the largest selection in this category. Ideally, you should have a good feel for the ground through the sole of the shoe. Consider this: The closer you get to being barefoot, the better for your feet and your forefoot step. Light footwear in itself is a plus. Without being flat and having ample toe space, however, such shoes are of little value.

Of course, there is also a vast array of other criteria, from price to production and from quality to style. All these factors play a minor role, however, compared to the aspects of flatness, toe space and weight.

And one final request: Please do not wear slippers or flip-flops! It is in the nature of things that shoes that provide no support to your heels will slip off your foot when you let it hang downward before taking a step. To avoid this, you have to "clutch" the shoe with your toes in order to hold it on your foot. This not only hinders a correct forefoot step, but additionally provokes tension in your feet and legs, which you can surely do without. You should also keep in mind that your feet need the stimuli they get from the ground to maintain healthy arches and a muscular balance. You lose the stimuli if you pack up your feet in inflexible shoes that also have a thick sole and are padded with various shock-absorbing systems or insoles. No stimulus, no tone. You will already know this if you've ever been unfortunate enough to get a cast put on your foot. So if you wear such footwear you shouldn't be surprised if you have flat feet or the structure of your feet is otherwise degenerated.

Last but not least …

And on this note I will let you loose into the wild to put everything into practice. I wish you all the best and hope you have fun with your feet and the forefoot step. Maybe one day we will meet in person at one of my forefoot step seminars. I would be happy to hear from you with feedback, suggestions or questions in a brief e-mail.
Just visit my blog at www.einfachballengang.de – which also has a "For international visitors" section – and stay in touch.

Best regards,

Dirk Beckmann

About the author

Dirk Beckmann is the most well-known expert in his field in the metropolitan area of Düsseldorf, Germany. Since 2005, he has worked with numerous clients in his own practice in Düsseldorf as a fascia therapist and specialist of body posture and functional gait patterns. His clients come from all over Germany as well as neighboring countries.
In addition to the manual treatment of myofascial adhesions he focuses on teaching and coaching functional movement patterns. Part of this includes the forefoot step, which Dirk Beckmann has already taught to hundreds of people in individual and group courses. Additionally, he is the author of a blog for "forefoot steppers" at www.einfachballengang.de, where he provides information to clients and anyone interested about this exciting topic – his busy schedule permitting, of course.